Vegetarian Food For Beginners

A Beginners's Guide To Cooking Healthy And Tasty Vegetarian Meals

Brigitte S. Romero

Vegetarian Food For Beginners

© Copyright 2021 - All rights reserved.

The content contained within this book may not be reproduced, duplicated or transmitted without direct written permission from the author or the publisher.

Under no circumstances will any blame or legal responsibility be held against the publisher, or author, for any damages, reparation, or monetary loss due to the information contained within this book. Either directly or indirectly.

Legal Notice:

This book is copyright protected. This book is only for personal use. You cannot amend, distribute, sell, use, quote or paraphrase any part, or the content within this book, without the consent of the author or publisher.

Disclaimer Notice:

Please note the information contained within this document is for educational and entertainment purposes only. All effort has been executed to present accurate, up to date, and reliable, complete information. No warranties of any kind are declared or implied. Readers acknowledge that the author is not engaging in the rendering of legal, financial, medical or professional advice. The content within this book has been derived from various sources. Please consult a licensed professional before attempting any techniques outlined in this book.

By reading this document, the reader agrees that under no circumstances is the author responsible for any losses, direct or indirect, which are incurred as a result of the use of information contained within this document, including, but not limited to, errors, omissions, or inaccuracies.

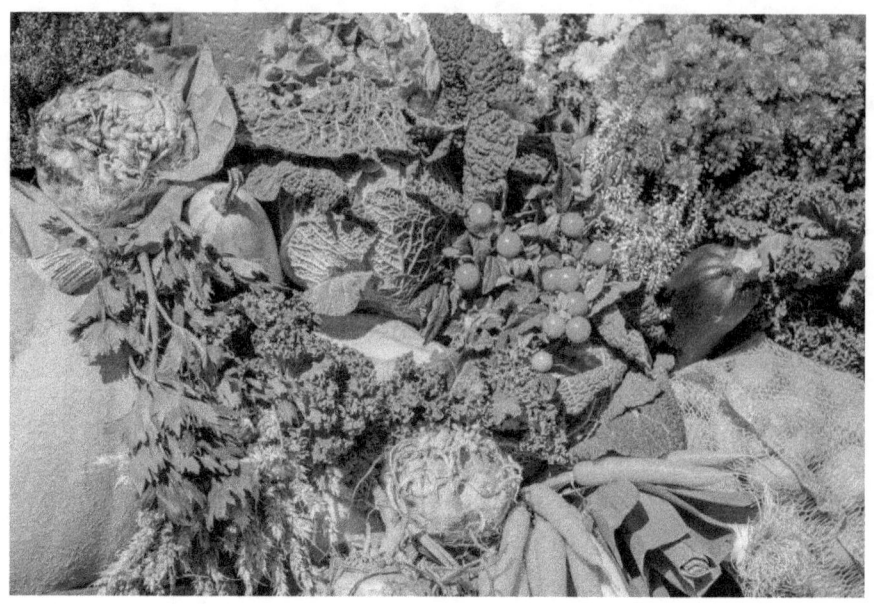

TABLE OF CONTENTS

INTRODUCTION **8**

CHAPTER 1: BREAKFAST RECIPES **12**

1. Mexican Breakfast Burritos 13
2. Scrambled Eggs 15
3. Spinach Feta Quiche 17
4. Raspberry Lemon Yogurt Parfaits 19
5. Peanut Butter Banana Smoothie 21
6. The Runner's Drink 23
7. Blueberry and Grape Brainiac Smoothie 24

CHAPTER 2: LUNCH RECIPES **26**

8. Roasted Jalapeño and Lime Guacamole 27
9. Avo-Tomato-Pasta 29
10. Braised Cabbage 31

CHAPTER 3: MAIN MEALS RECIPES **32**

11. Tempeh Split Pea Burgers 33
12. Crispy Marinated Tempeh 35
13. BBQ-LT Sandwich 37

CHAPTER 4: VEGETABLES, SALADS AND SIDES RECIPES **40**

14. Brussels Sprout Salad 41
15. Instant Sweet Potato 43
16. Maple-glazed Brussels sprouts 45
17. Spaghetti Squash 46
18. Flavorful Roasted Peppers 48
19. Spicy Cajun Boiled Peanuts 49
20. Savory Squash & Apple Dish 50

CHAPTER 5: DESSERT RECIPES 52

- 21. VEGAN WHIPPED CREAM 52
- 22. PATTY'S THREE-MINUTE FUDGE 54
- 23. HEALTHY AVOCADO CHOCOLATE PUDDING 56

CHAPTER 6: SNACK RECIPES 58

- 24. RAW STRAWBERRY CRUMBLE 58
- 25. PEANUT BUTTER ENERGY BARS 60
- 26. SUNFLOWER PARMESAN "CHEESE" 62
- 27. BANANA PEANUT BUTTER YOGURT BOWL 63
- 28. PEANUT BUTTER FUDGE 64
- 29. ROASTED CHICKPEAS 65
- 30. TAMARI ALMONDS 67
- 31. TACO PITA PIZZAS 69
- 32. RISOTTO BITES 71
- 33. HEALTHY PROTEIN BARS 73

CHAPTER 7: JUICES AND SMOOTHIES RECIPES 76

- 34. MANGO SMOOTHIE 76
- 35. BEETROOT SMOOTHIE 78
- 36. AVOCADO SMOOTHIE 79
- 37. RED SMOOTHIE 80
- 38. KALE SMOOTHIE 81
- 39. MELON SMOOTHIE 82

CHAPTER 8: OTHER RECIPES 84

- 40. CAULIFLOWER MASH 84
- 41. APPLE LEATHER 86
- 42. SAUTÉED BRUSSELS SPROUT 88
- 43. GREEN BEANS WITH MUSHROOMS 90
- 44. PINTO BEANS WITH SALSA 92

45.	ASPARAGUS SOUP	94
46.	BEET SOUP	96
47.	PEARS IN RED WINE SAUCE	97
48.	POLENTA	98
49.	CARROTS IN THYME	100
50.	SMOKY PECAN BRUSSELS SPROUTS	101

CONCLUSION **104**

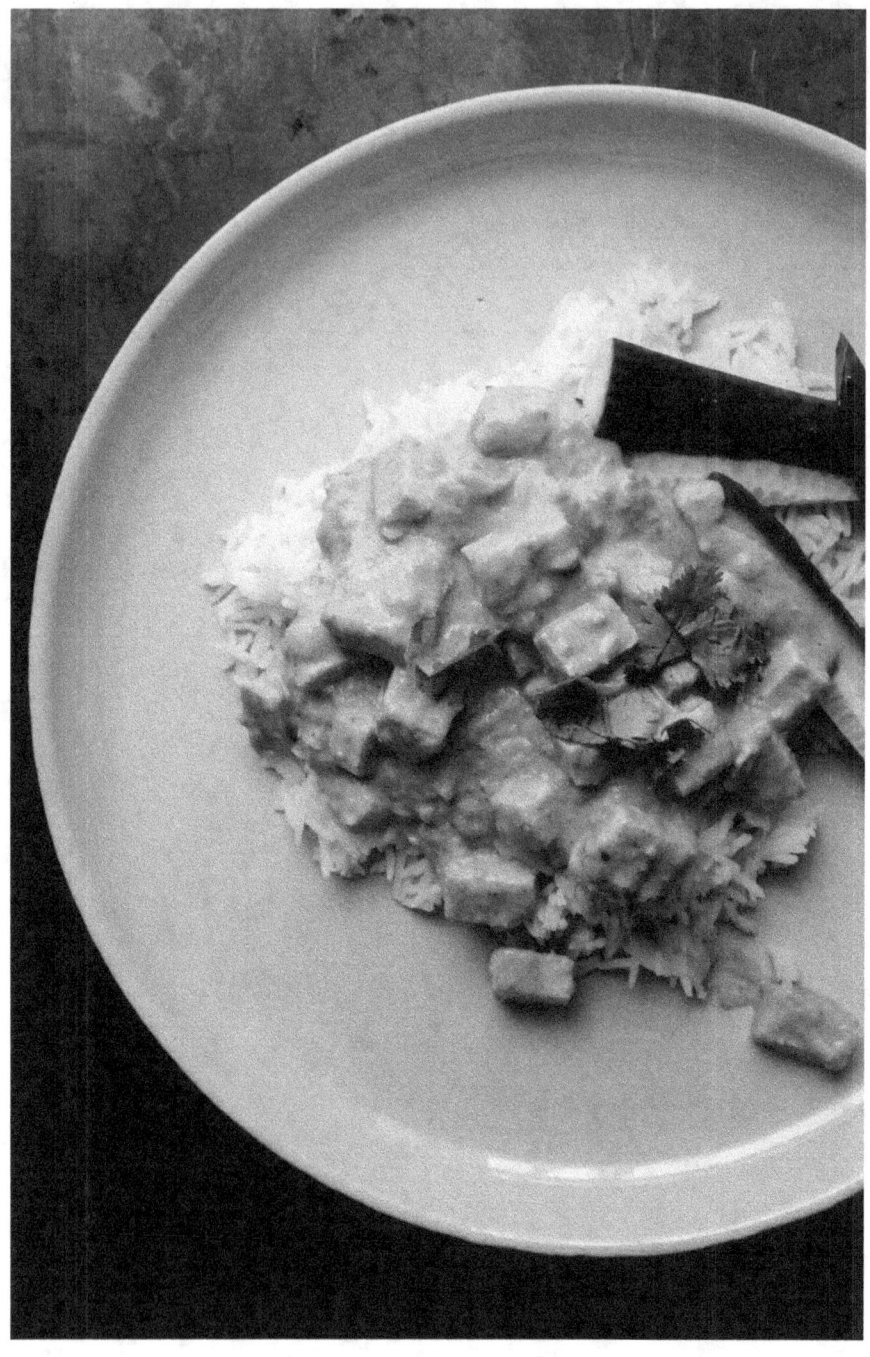

INTRODUCTION

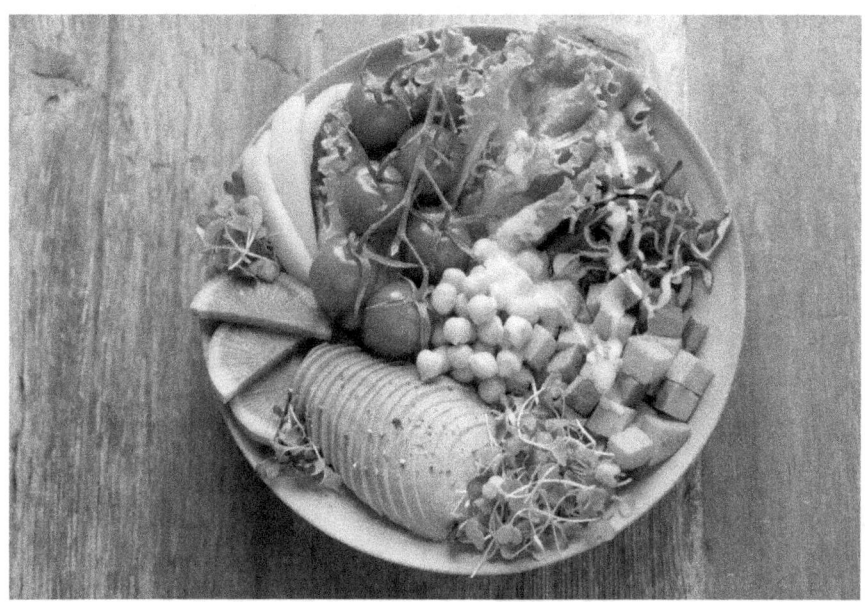

Vegetarianism is not a new concept; it has been practiced since ancient times in India during the Vedic period (1500-500 BC) as well as in Greece and Rome. It continues to be practiced today in modern society around the world. In most cases, it is a matter of individual choice.

Eating meat and fish has been a common practice all over the world for thousands of years. In some cultures, the preparation of the meat or fish symbolizes wealth and luxury, while in others it represents a source of survival. Today, people are becoming more aware of the impact that their food choices have on their health as well as on the environment.

Why do people become vegetarians? The reasons vary widely from person to person. Some people object to the cruelty and suffering of animals raised for food. Some people object to the environmental effects of producing meat and fish. Others become vegetarians because they believe animal flesh is unhealthy to eat or because they believe it is unspiritual or unwise. For some, it is a choice of economic necessity.

How often should you eat fruits and vegetables? The recommendation is to eat five servings per day based on a 2,000 calorie diet. One serving is equal to one-half cup raw or one cup ready-to-eat. Fruits and vegetables provide vitamins, minerals, fiber, and other nutrients that are essential for good health. It is recommended that most Americans make fruits and vegetables the basis of their diet; ideally, they should be eaten at every meal.

So, specifically, what are the foods that one needs to avoid? These are as follows:

- Beef
- Pork
- Lamb
- Veal
- All Game (deer, elk, etc.)
- Any other land mammal that's been fed animal products or by-products such as eggs and dairy (many land mammals are herbivores)
- Fish and Shellfish
- Goose and Duck
- Emu and Alligator
- Any other animal that is not a seafood product
- Animal by-products such as gelatin (e.g., gummy bears)

As a vegetarian, what specific foods do you avoid? For starters, you can limit your consumption of the following:

- Pork and bacon
- Eggs (or eat only eggs that are certified organic or non-cage free)
- Dairy products (or consume only dairy products that are certified organic)
- All products that are made from animals, such as leather shoes, belts, jackets, etc.

What are the substitutes that you use to replace the meat and fish that you avoid?

- Tofu (made from soybeans)
- Tempeh (made from soybeans)
- TVP (textured vegetable protein)
- Seitan (very high in protein, available as steak strips or chicken-style pieces)
- Soy Nuggets/Sausage

Being a vegetarian has its benefits, but there are definitely some challenges as well. If you are considering the option of being a vegetarian, the most important thing to consider is your overall health. However, if you have concerns with the lack of protein in your diet, believe that it's unwise to eat only plant products, or simply crave meat and fish and think you can't give them up without feeling hungry or deprived, then the choice of becoming a vegetarian may not be the right one for you.

This vegetarian cookbook will help you get a delicious and healthy recipe on the table that will make your life less stressful. A good recipe doesn't need a long list of ingredients to make it tasty, and while preparing meals may seem hard. You can eat together a healthy family food in the same amount of time you'd need to order takeout!

This vegetarian cookbook will show you a variety of dishes you can make with easy-to-find ingredients. This is the perfect practical guide for anyone looking to make a variety of delicious meals that are healthy. It includes recipes for breakfast, lunch, dinner, appetizers, and desserts, as well as those for snacks and sides. Whether looking to lose weight or just eat more healthily, this cookbook will make it easier than ever before!

So, let us begin the journey.

CHAPTER 1:

BREAKFAST RECIPES

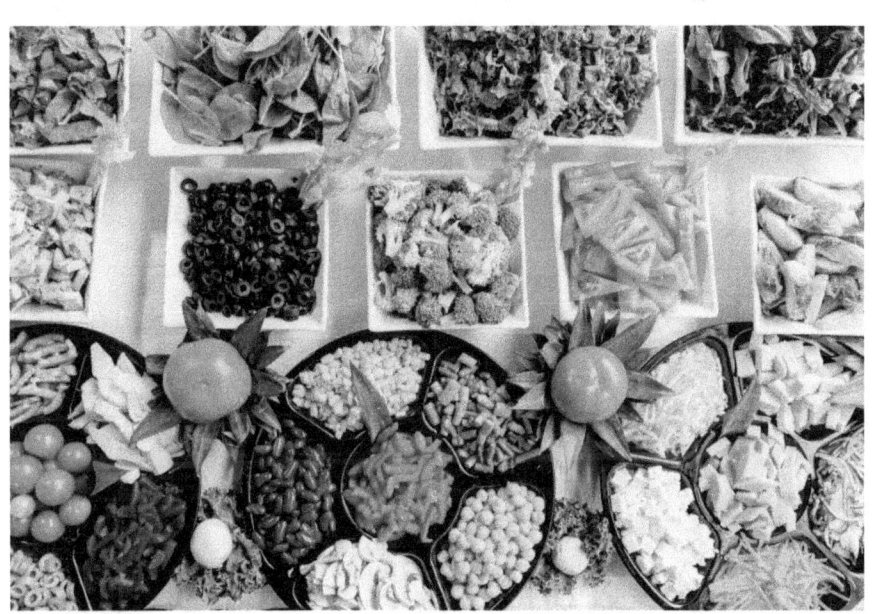

1. Mexican Breakfast Burritos

Preparation Time: 10 minutes

Cooking Time: 5 minutes

Servings: 6

Ingredients:

- 1 batch Perfect Scrambled Eggs
- 1 cup canned black beans, rinsed
- 1 cup shredded Cheddar cheese
- 6 (10- to 12-inch) flour tortillas
- ¾ cup Three-Minute Blender Salsa or your favorite jarred salsa, plus more for serving
- Optional: Sour cream and guacamole for serving

Directions:

1. Follow the recipe for Perfect Scrambled Eggs. Stir in the beans and cheese in the last 2 minutes of cooking.
2. Warm the tortillas in the microwave for about 10 seconds, so they are pliable.

3. Add some of the egg filling to the center of each tortilla. Top with a few spoonfuls of salsa. Wrap the burritos tightly. Serve and enjoy!

Nutrition: Calories: 147 Carbs: 8g Fat: 4g Protein: 10g

2. Scrambled Eggs

Preparation Time: 5 minutes

Cooking Time: 5 minutes

Servings: 4

Ingredients:

- 8 large eggs
- ½ teaspoon salt, plus more for seasoning
- 2 tablespoons water
- 2 tablespoons salted butter
- Black pepper

Directions:

1. Crack eggs into a bowl and whisk rapidly with salt and water for 30 seconds, or until the eggs are blended together and start to foam.

2. Melt the butter on low heat in a medium nonstick skillet. When the butter bubbles, add egg mixture to the pan.

3. The eggs will start to cook in about 30 seconds. As they begin to get firm around the edges of the pan, use a heatproof rubber spatula to push them to the center of the pan. Stir as the eggs form large curds—soft but solid pieces of boiled egg within the liquid egg mixture. Remove the pan from the stove when all the eggs are firm but still soft and no visible liquid remains. Cooking should be about 2 to 3 minutes.

4. Season with salt and pepper to taste.

5. Technique Tutorial: Whisking the eggs incorporates air into them, so the more muscle you use in whisking, the lighter and fluffier the eggs will be.

Nutrition: Calories: 295 Carbs: 9g Fat: 21g Protein: 19g

3. Spinach Feta Quiche

Preparation Time: 10 minutes

Cooking Time: 50 minutes

Servings: 6

Ingredients:

- 10-ounce package frozen spinach
- 1 cup whole milk
- 5 large eggs
- 6 ounces crumbled feta cheese with Mediterranean herbs (or plain)
- 1 refrigerated pie crust, brought to room temperature

Directions:

1. Preheat the oven to 350°F.
2. Drain all the water and squeeze out of the spinach. You can use a colander for this.
3. In a bowl, mix the spinach, milk, eggs, and cheese.

4. Unroll pie crust and then press it into a 9- to 10-inch pie plate. Crimp the edges with a fork (press the ends of the fork tines down on the rim, making sure to go around the whole rim) and make sure the pie crust is uniform all around the rim.

5. Pour egg in the pie crust, making sure not to overfill.

6. Bake it for 45-50 minutes until the quiche is set. Make sure the crust is golden brown around the edges. Poke it using a toothpick. To know that this is already done, it should come out clean.

7. Cool for 10 to 20 minutes before serving.

8. Simple Swap: If you prefer, use 10 ounces of fresh baby spinach in place of frozen spinach. Chop it and sauté. Pour olive oil into a skillet and put it on medium-high heat until wilted. The idea is to cook it until most of the water is removed. It can then be added to the egg mixture in step 3.

Nutrition: Calories: 141 Carbs: 9g Fat: 9g Protein: 7g

4. **Raspberry Lemon Yogurt Parfaits**

Preparation Time: 5 minutes

Cooking Time: 0 minutes

Servings: 4

Ingredients:

- 2 cups raspberries, plus 4 extra raspberries, for garnish
- 4 (6-ounce) containers lemon yogurt
- ½ cup granola
- 2 tablespoons sliced or chopped almonds

Directions:

1. Divide the raspberries evenly into four parfait glasses. Top each with half a container of yogurt.
2. Sprinkle each with granola. Top with the remaining yogurt. Sprinkle the almonds on top.
3. Garnish with the extra raspberries and serve.
4. Prep Tip: If you do not have parfait glasses, you can use cocktail or highball glasses. Small mason jars work too. It won't really

matter what you put the parfaits in because as soon as you serve them, they will disappear.

Nutrition: Calories: 168 Carbs: 30g Fat: 3g Protein: 5g

5. **Peanut Butter Banana Smoothie**

Preparation Time: 5 minutes

Cooking Time: 0 minutes

Servings: 4

Ingredients:

- 4 small frozen ripe bananas, peeled and sliced
- 2 cups 2% milk
- 8 ounces vanilla Greek yogurt
- ¼ cup smooth peanut butter
- 1 cup ice

Directions:

1. Add the bananas, milk, yogurt, peanut butter, and ice to a blender. Blend it for 2-3 minutes, or until the mixture is smooth.

2. If you don't have a blender, put all the ingredients in a large bowl and using an electric mixer until all lumps are gone at low speed. If the mixture is smooth, but large pieces of ice remain, just pick

them out with a spoon before transferring the smoothies to glasses.

3. Serve in tall glasses with straws.

4. Prep Tip: To store bananas in the freezer, peel and slice the bananas and seal each banana individually in a small freezer bag. Take them out when ready to use.

Nutrition: Calories: 229 Carbs: 31g Fat: 10g Protein: 7g

6. The Runner's Drink

Preparation Time: 10 minutes

Cooking Time: 0 minutes

Servings: 1

Ingredients:

- 2 teaspoons chia seeds
- 1¼ cups water
- Juice of 1 lemon or lime
- Drizzle of pure maple syrup

Directions:

1. Shake or stir together the chia seeds, water, and citrus juice. Sweeten with a drizzle of maple syrup.
2. Pour over ice and serve.
3. Substitution Tip: Add ¼ cup of frozen berries for a more tropical drink. Let them sit for 30 minutes to defrost before adding to the drink.

Nutrition: Calories: 84 Fat: 4g Carbohydrate: 10g Protein: 2g

7. Blueberry and Grape Brainiac Smoothie

Preparation Time: 5 minutes

Cooking Time: 0 minutes

Servings: 4

Ingredients:

- 2 cups blueberries
- 2 cups seedless red or black grapes
- 4 cups unsweetened almond milk
- 2 tablespoons pure maple syrup
- 4 tablespoons ground flaxseed
- 1 cup ice cubes

Directions:

1. In a blender or food processor, purée everything together until smooth.

2. Ingredient Tip: Smoothie recipes are surprisingly simple to make and customize. Just remember this simple formula: fruit + nondairy milk + healthy fat like nuts, avocado, or seeds + ice.

Optional add-ins include leafy greens for iron and folate, one frozen banana for extra potassium and vitamin C, a sweetener like a maple syrup, and a sugar-free protein powder.

Nutrition: Calories: 242 Fat: 11g Carbohydrate: 32g Protein: 6g

CHAPTER 2:

LUNCH RECIPES

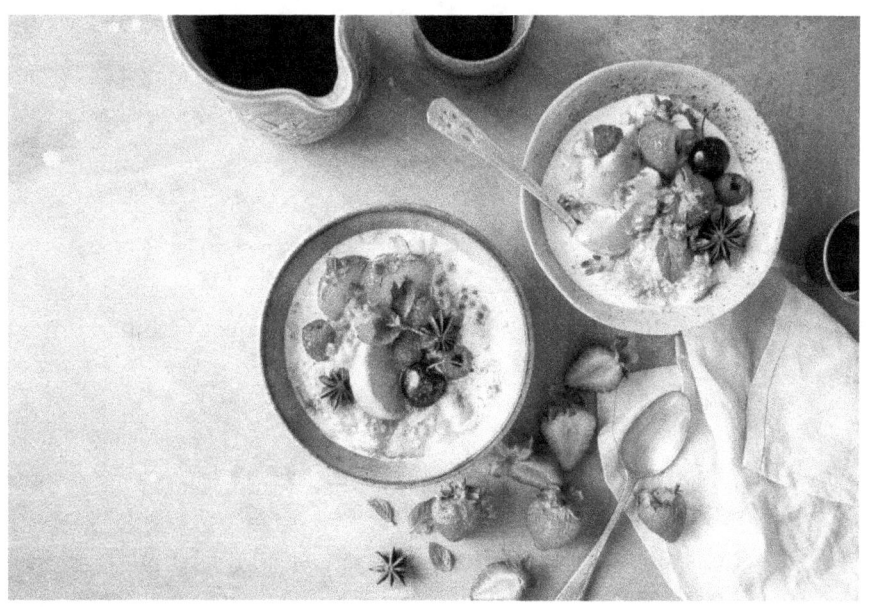

8. Roasted Jalapeño and Lime Guacamole

Preparation Time: 5 minutes

Cooking Time: 10 minutes

Servings: 4

Ingredients:

- 1 to 3 jalapeños (depending on your preferred level of spiciness)
- 1 avocado, peeled and pitted
- 1 tablespoon freshly squeezed lime juice

Directions:

1. Preheat the oven to 400°F. Line a baking sheet with parchment paper.
2. Place the jalapeños on the baking sheet and roast for 8 minutes. (The jalapeño can also be roasted on a grill for 5 minutes if you already have it fired up.)
3. Slice the jalapeños and remove the seeds. Cut the top stem and dice into ⅛-inch pieces. Wash your hands immediately after handling the jalapeños.

4. Use a fork or a masher to mash together the avocado, jalapeño pieces, and lime juice and in a medium bowl. Mash and mix until the guacamole has the preferred consistency. Then serve and enjoy!

Nutrition: Calories: 77 Total fat: 7g Carbohydrates: 5g Fiber: 3g Protein: 1g

9. Avo-Tomato-Pasta

Preparation Time: 5 minutes

Cooking Time: 10 minutes

Servings: 4

Ingredients:

- 7 oz. pasta
- 1 diced avocado
- 14 oz. cherry tomatoes halved or quartered
- 4 tbsp. vinaigrette
- 1 clove garlic 7

Directions:

1. Cook pasta base on the instructions of the packaging. Add the garlic to infuse the taste.

2. Drain the pasta slowly and remove the garlic. In a bowl, mix the avocado and tomatoes, and lightly toss in the vinaigrette. Mash the garlic and add it to the avocado mixture.

3. Drizzle a little olive oil all over the pasta. Mix the avocado mixture into the pasta and serve immediately.

Nutrition: Calories: 371 Total fat: 51g Carbohydrates: 11g Fiber: 16g

10. Braised Cabbage

Preparation Time: 10 minutes

Cooking Time: 10 minutes

Servings: 3

Ingredients:

- 14 oz. chopped cabbage
- 1 onion cut into rings
- 2 peeled and diced tomatoes
- Olive oil for cooking

Directions:

1. Put olive oil in a frying pan and turn it over medium heat. Sauté the onion rings for 3 minutes until soft and starting to brown.
2. Add the tomatoes and braise for another 3 minutes. Reduce the heat and add the cabbage. Stir fry for another 4 minutes until the cabbage softens.
3. Serve while still warm.

Nutrition: Calories: 90 Total fat: 20g Carbohydrates: 1g Fiber: 1g

CHAPTER 3:

MAIN MEALS RECIPES

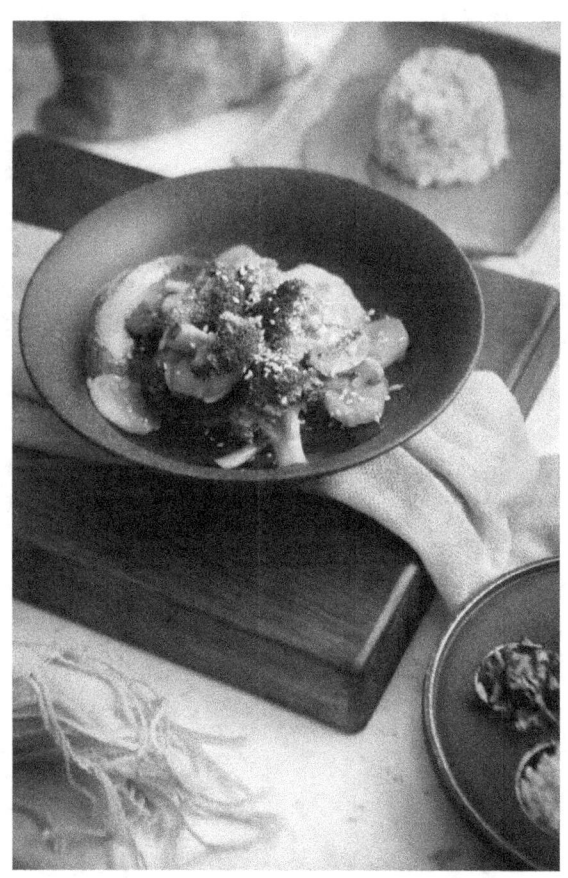

11. Tempeh Split Pea Burgers

Preparation Time: 10 minutes

Cooking Time: 25 minutes

Servings: 8

Ingredients:

- 3 cups Split peas (cooked or canned)
- 1 14-ounces pack Tempeh
- ½ cup Full-fat coconut milk
- 3 tablespoons Ground flaxseeds
- 3 tablespoons Burger spices

Directions:

1. Cook dry split peas, soak and cook 1 cup (200 g.) of dry split peas according to the procedure in the package.
2. Preheat the oven to 350°F. Line a baking sheet using parchment paper.

3. Add tempeh to the food processor and blend it until a chunky mixture is achieved. Scrape down the sides of the food processor to prevent any lumps.

4. Add the split peas, ground flaxseed, and spices to the food processor and slowly process it along with the tempeh while pouring in the coconut milk to form a chunky mixture.

5. You can also crumble the tempeh by hand in a large bowl, add the remaining ingredients, and mash everything into a chunky mixture.

6. Put every mixture on the baking sheet. Make sure to flatten it into a 1-inch thick. Cut it in square patties making 8 pieces. You can also shape each patty into a circle before baking.

7. Bake the patties for 15 minutes. Take the baking sheet off the oven, then flip the patties. Bake again for another 10 minutes.

8. Take patties out of the oven once the crust is crispy and browned and let them cool down for about a minute.

9. Serve and enjoy!

Nutrition: Calories: 236 Carbs: 18 g. Fat: 9.5 g. Protein: 18.3 g.

12. Crispy Marinated Tempeh

Preparation Time: 15 minutes

Cooking Time: 25 minutes

Servings: 2

Ingredients:

- 1 14-ounces pack Tempeh (cubed)
- ¼ cup Low-sodium soy sauce
- ¼ cup Lemon juice
- 4-inches piece Ginger (minced)
- 4 cloves Garlic (minced)

Directions:

1. Put the tempeh cubes in an airtight with all the other ingredients.
2. Close and shake well until the tempeh cubes are covered evenly with the ingredients.
3. Use an airtight container and put it in the fridge for at least 2 hours or overnight to make sure the tempeh is marinated thoroughly.

4. Preheat oven to 375°F. Line a baking sheet using parchment paper.

5. Transfer tempeh onto the baking sheet, then bake for 25 minutes or until the tempeh is browned and crispy.

6. Serve the tempeh and enjoy!

Nutrition: Calories: 431 Carbs: 10.5 g. Fat: 19.4 g. Protein: 47.9 g

13. **BBQ-LT Sandwich**

Preparation Time: 15 minutes

Cooking Time: 15 minutes

Servings: 2

Ingredients:

- 1 7-ounces pack Tempeh (thinly sliced)
- ½ cup BBQ sauce
- 2 large tomatoes (sliced)
- 4 leaves Lettuce
- 4 whole wheat buns

Directions:

1. Add the tempeh slices and the BBQ sauce to an airtight container.
2. Close airtight container, mix well and put it in the fridge. Allow the tempeh to marinate for 1 hour up until 12 hours.
3. Preheat your oven to 375°F. Line a baking sheet u parchment paper.

4. Transfer the tempeh slices onto the baking sheet and bake for about 15 minutes or until the tempeh is browned and crispy.

5. Bake the buns with the tempeh for the last 5 minutes if you want crispy and browned bread.

6. Spread the optional guacamole on the bottom half of each bun and add a lettuce leaf on top,

7. Put a quarter of the BBQ tempeh slices on top of the lettuce on each bun. Top it with 2 slices of tomato per bun.

8. Cover with the top halves of the buns, serve the sandwiches right away, and enjoy!

Nutrition: Calories: 260 Carbs: 14.85 g. Fat: 10 g. Protein: 24 g.

CHAPTER 4:

VEGETABLES, SALADS AND SIDES RECIPES

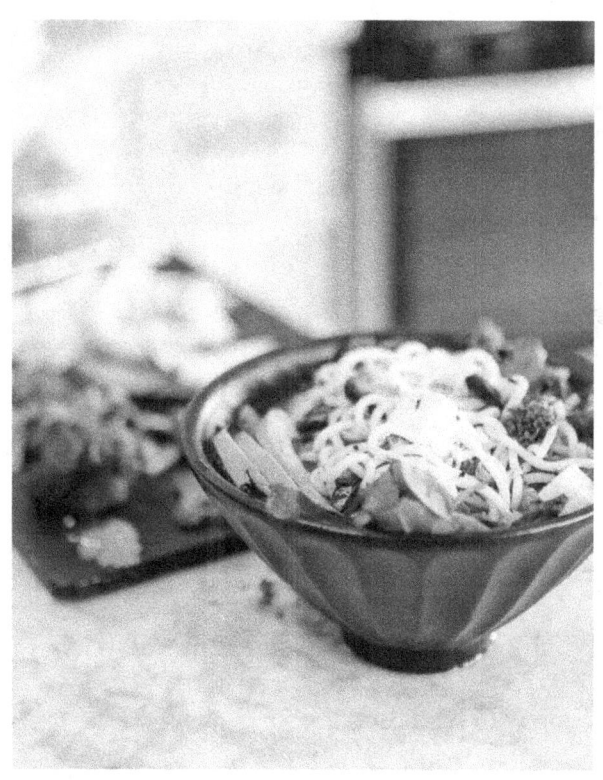

14. Brussels Sprout Salad

Preparation Time: 5 minutes

Cooking Time: 5 minutes

Servings: 8

Ingredients:

- 2 lbs. Brussels sprouts, trimmed and halved
- 1 tablespoon unsalted butter, melted
- 1 cup water
- 2 cups pomegranate seeds
- ½ cup almonds, chopped

Directions:

1. Put some water into the insert of Instant Pot.
2. Place the steamer trivet inside.
3. Arrange the Brussels sprouts over the trivet.
4. Make sure that the lid is close tightly and select the "Manual" function with high pressure for 5 minutes.
5. After the beep, do a Natural release and remove the lid.

6. Transfer the sprouts to a platter and pour melted butter on top.

7. Sprinkle almonds and pomegranate seeds on top and serve.

Nutrition: Calories: 196 Carbohydrate: 35.6g Protein: 5.1g Fat: 4.8g

15. Instant Sweet Potato

Preparation Time: 5 minutes

Cooking Time: 10 minutes

Servings: 2

Ingredients:

- 1 cup water
- 2 medium sweet potatoes, peeled
- Salt and pepper to taste
- 1 tablespoon olive oil
- 2 tablespoons chopped fresh parsley to garnish
- Pomegranate seeds as needed to garnish

Directions:

1. Put some water into the insert of Instant Pot.
2. Place the steamer trivet inside.
3. Arrange the sweet potatoes over the trivet.
4. Secure the lid and select the "Steam" function for 10 minutes.

5. After the beep, do a Natural release and remove the lid.

6. Remove the potatoes and cut them into cubes.

7. Add oil and potatoes into the Instant Pot and "Sauté" for 5 minutes while stirring.

8. Garnish with parsley and pomegranate seeds.

9. Serve

Nutrition: Calories: 100 Carbohydrate: 23g Protein: 2g Fat: 0g

16. Maple-glazed Brussels sprouts

Preparation Time: 10 minutes Cooking Time: 4 minutes

Servings: 4

Ingredients:

- 1 lb. Brussels sprouts (trimmed)
- 2 tablespoons freshly squeezed orange juice
- ½ teaspoon grated orange zest
- ½ tablespoon Earth Balance buttery spread
- 1 tablespoon maple syrup
- Salt and black pepper to taste

Directions:

1. Put all the ingredients in the Instant Pot.
2. Make sure that the lid is closed tightly and select the "Manual" function for 4 minutes with high pressure.
3. Do a quick release after the beep and then remove the lid.
4. Stir well and serve immediately.

Nutrition: Calories: 166 Carbohydrate: 14.5g Protein: 3.9g Fat: 11.4g

17. Spaghetti Squash

Preparation Time: 5 minutes

Cooking Time: 20 minutes

Servings: 2

Ingredients:

- 1 (2 lbs.) spaghetti squash
- 1 cup water
- 2 tablespoons fresh cilantro to garnish (optional)

Directions:

1. Slice the squash in half. Remove the seeds from its center.
2. Put some water into the insert of Instant Pot and place the trivet inside.
3. Arrange two halves of the squash over the trivet, with the skin side down.
4. Secure the lid and select "Manual" with high pressure for 20 minutes.
5. After the beep, do a Natural release and remove the lid.

6. Remove the squash and use two forks to shred it from inside.

7. Serve with fresh cilantro.

Nutrition: Calories: 146 Carbohydrate: 32.2g Protein: 3.4g Fat: 2.6g

18. Flavorful Roasted Peppers

Preparation Time: 2 minutes Cooking Time: 3 hours 20 minutes

Servings: 5

Ingredients:

- 5 medium-sized red bell pepper, cored and halved

Directions:

1. Take a 6-quarts slow cooker, grease it with a non-stick cooking spray and add the peppers.
2. Cover the top, plug in the slow cooker; adjust the cooking time to 3 hours and let it cook on the high heat setting or until the peppers are softened, stirring halfway through.
3. When done, remove the peppers from the cooker and let them cool off completely.
4. Then remove the pepper peels by tugging them from the edge or with a paring knife.
5. Serve as desired.

Nutrition: Calories: 5 Carbohydrates: 1g Protein: 0g Fats: 0g

19. Spicy Cajun Boiled Peanuts

Preparation Time: 5 minutes Cooking Time: 8 hours

Servings: 15

Ingredients:

- 5 pounds of peanuts, raw and in shells
- 6-ounce of dry crab boil
- 4-ounce of jalapeno peppers, sliced
- 2-ounce of vegetable broth

Directions:

1. Take a 6-quarts slow cooker, place the ingredients in it, and cover it with water.
2. Stir properly and cover the top.
3. Plug in the slow cooker; adjust the cooking time to 8 hours and let it cook on the low heat setting or until the peanuts are soft and floats on top of the cooking liquid.
4. Drain the nuts and serve right away.

Nutrition: Calories: 309 Carbohydrates: 5g Protein: 0g

20. Savory Squash & Apple Dish

Preparation Time: 10 minutes

Cooking Time: 4 hours 15 minutes

Servings: 6

Ingredients:

- 8 ounce of dried cranberries
- 4 medium-sized apples, peeled, cored and chopped
- 3 pounds of butternut squash, peeled, seeded and cubed
- Half of a medium-sized white onion, peeled and diced
- 1 tablespoon of ground cinnamon
- 1 1/2 teaspoons of ground nutmeg

Directions:

1. Take a 6-quarts slow cooker, grease it with a non-stick cooking spray, and place the ingredients in it.
2. Stir properly and cover the top.
3. Plug in the slow cooker; adjust the cooking time to 4 hours and let it cook on the low heat setting or until it cooks thoroughly.

4. Serve right away.

Nutrition: Calories: 210 Carbohydrates: 11g Protein: 3g Fats: 5g

CHAPTER 5:

DESSERT RECIPES

21. Vegan Whipped Cream

Preparation Time: 10 minutes

Cooking Time: 0 minutes

Servings: 2

Ingredients:

- 1 (13- to 14-ounce) can unsweetened, full-fat coconut milk
- 3 teaspoons sugar or any vegan sweetener
- 1 teaspoon pure vanilla extract

Directions:

1. Put the can of full-fat coconut milk overnight in the refrigerator.

2. Place it in a large metal bowl and electric beaters from an electric hand mixer in the freezer for an hour, then prepare the whipped cream.

3. Open a cold can of coconut milk (make sure to not shake it). The coconut cream solids will have hardened on the top. Spoon just the solids into the cold mixing bowl, avoiding the liquid.

4. Use an electric mixer in mixing coconut cream until stiff peaks form.

5. Then add sugar and vanilla, then beat another minute. Taste and add more sweetener if needed.

6. Leftovers: This whipped cream will stay fresh for 3 to 5 days in a sealed container in the refrigerator.

Nutrition: Calories: 41 Fat: 2g Carbohydrate: 6g Protein: 0g

22. Patty's Three-Minute Fudge

Preparation Time: 10 minutes

Cooking Time: 0 minutes

Servings: 6

Ingredients:

- Vegan butter
- 2 cups dark semisweet vegan chocolate chips
- 1 (14.5-ounce) can vegan sweetened condensed milk
- 1 teaspoon vanilla extract

Directions:

1. Grease an 8-inch square pan with vegan butter and line with parchment paper.

2. In a microwave-safe two-quart bowl, heat the chocolate chips and condensed milk on high for 1 minute. Let rest for a minute, then stir to combine. If needed, heat an additional 30 seconds. Stir until completely melted and the chocolate is smooth. Stir in the vanilla.

3. Pour the fudge into the prepared pan. Make it cool and set for about 1 hour. Then cut into squares.

4. The fudge will keep at room temperature, covered, for 1 to 2 days.

Nutrition: Calories: 89 Fat: 4g Carbohydrate: 12g Protein: 1g

23. Healthy Avocado Chocolate Pudding

Preparation Time: 5 minutes

Cooking Time: 0 minutes

Servings: 4

Ingredients:

- 6 avocados, peeled, pitted, and cut into chunks
- ½ cup pure maple syrup, or more to taste
- ¾ cup unsweetened cocoa powder
- 2 teaspoons vanilla extract
- Fresh mint leaves, optional

Directions:

1. In a food processor, purée the avocados, maple syrup, cocoa powder, and vanilla until smooth.
2. Garnish with mint leaves, if desired.
3. Ingredient Tip: Avoid leftovers and eat it all! The avocado will oxidize and turn brown after just a few hours.

Nutrition: Calories: 578 Fat: 42g Carbohydrate: 58g Protein: 8g

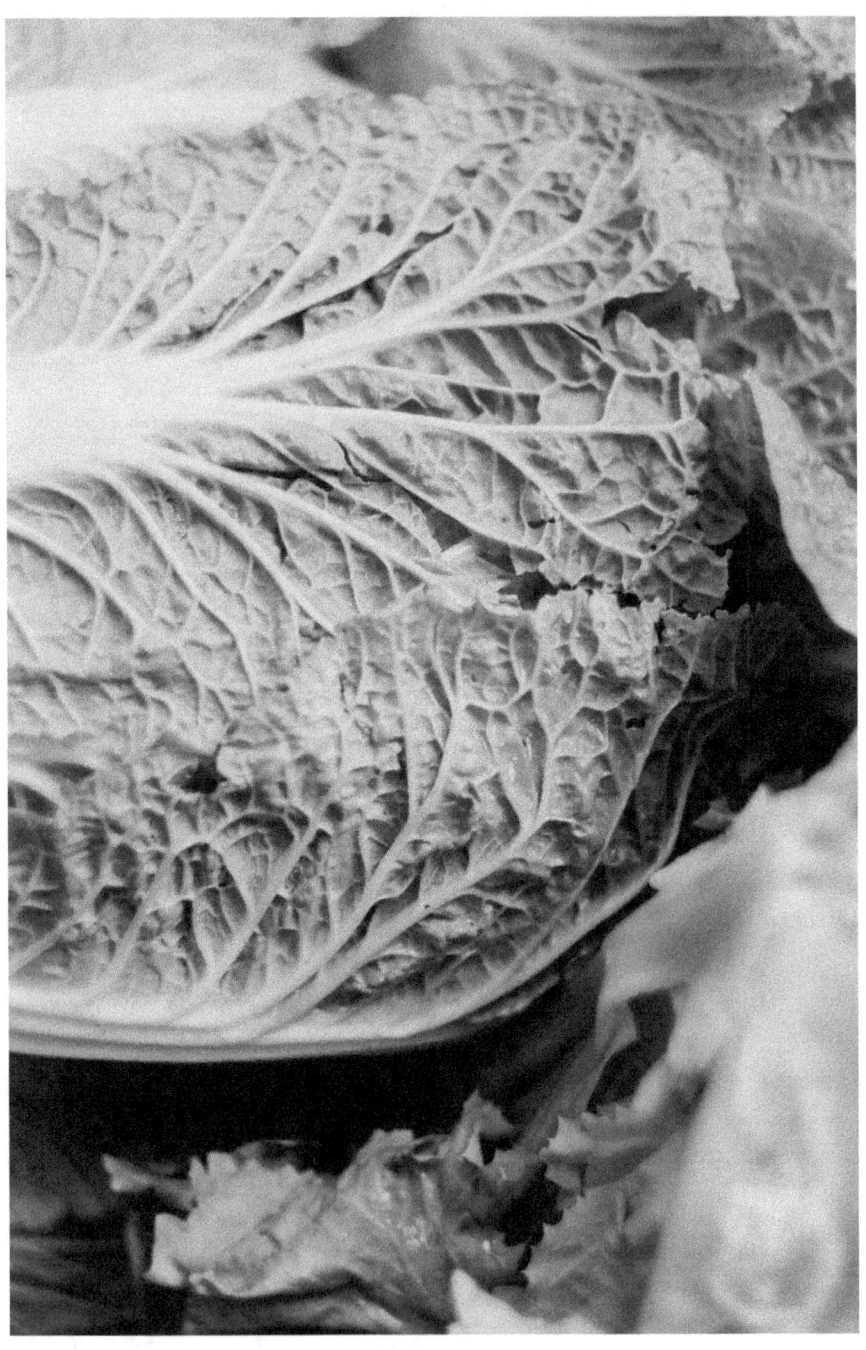

CHAPTER 6:

SNACK RECIPES

24. Raw Strawberry Crumble

Preparation Time: 10 minutes

Cooking Time: 5 minutes

Servings: 6

Ingredients:

- 4 cups fresh strawberries, hulled and sliced
- ¼ cup unsweetened coconut flakes
- ½ cup raw walnuts
- ½ tbsp. Ginger, grated
- ½ tbsp. ground cinnamon

Directions:

1. Arrange sliced strawberries on the bottom of a pie dish or serving bowls.

2. Add all of the rest of the ingredients to a food processor and pulse until a crumble consistency is.

3. Arrange the crumble on top of the strawberries and serve.

Nutrition: Fat: 15.7g Carbohydrates: 6.1g Protein: 13.1g

25. Peanut Butter Energy Bars

Preparation Time: 10 minutes

Cooking Time: 10 minutes

Servings: 8

Ingredients:

- 1 cup smooth peanut butter
- 4 teaspoons granulated erythritol
- ⅓ cup coconut flour
- 2 tablespoons water

Directions:

1. Get a 9-inch loaf pan and put a parchment paper.
2. Mix erythritol, peanut butter, and water in a medium bowl until a smooth consistency is achieved.
3. Stir in coconut flour and blend well to make a very thick but not dry mixture. If the mixture appears dry, add a few more teaspoons of water.
4. Press mixture into prepared loaf pan.

5. Put it in the refrigerator for at least 2 hours until set firm.

6. Remove the chilled bars from the loaf pan and cut them into bars. Serve. Can be stored in a tight container to refrigerate it up to 1 month or up to 6 months in the freezer.

Nutrition: Fat: 17g Carbohydrates: 13.8g Protein: 9.1g

26. Sunflower Parmesan "Cheese"

Preparation Time: 5 minutes

Cooking Time: 25 minutes

Servings: 4

Ingredients:

- ½ cup sunflower seeds
- 2 tablespoons nutritional yeast
- ½ teaspoon garlic powder

Directions:

1. Combine the sunflower seeds, nutritional yeast, and garlic powder in a food processor or blender. Process on low for 30 to 45 seconds, or until the sunflower seeds have been broken down into a chunk- like.

2. Store in a refrigerator-safe container for up to 2 months.

Nutrition: Calories: 56 Total fat: 4g Carbohydrates: 3g Fiber: 1g Protein: 3g

27. Banana Peanut Butter Yogurt Bowl

Preparation Time: 5 minutes

Cooking Time: 0 minutes

Servings: 4

Ingredients:

- 1 teaspoon nutmeg
- ¼ Creamy peanut butter
- 2 medium-sized sliced bananas
- 4 cups vanilla flavor
- Soy yogurt

Directions:

1. Divide the yogurt among four bowls and top with the slices of bananas. Soften the microwave in the microwave for forty seconds and then put one tablespoon into each bowl, then garnish with the nutmeg and flaxseed meal.

Nutrition: Calories 292 Fat 15g Carbs 24g Protein 29g Fiber 3g

28. Peanut Butter Fudge

Preparation Time: 30 minutes

Cooking Time: 0 minutes

Servings: 20

Ingredients:

- 1 teaspoon vanilla extract
- 3 tablespoons maple syrup
- ½ cup coconut oil
- 1 cup creamy peanut butter
- 2 cups coconut flakes, unsweetened

Directions:

1. Use spray oil on an eight-inch square pan. Cream the shredded coconut in a food processor until it forms a buttery substance. Put the coconut butter into a bowl and blend in the coconut oil and peanut butter. Then add in the vanilla and mix once more. Spoon the mix into the pan and let it set.

Nutrition: Calories 164 Protein 4g Fiber 2g Carbs 5g Fat 16g

29. Roasted Chickpeas

Preparation Time: 5 minutes

Cooking Time: 30 minutes

Servings: 4

Ingredients:

- 1 (14.5-ounce) can chickpeas, drained but not rinsed
- 1 teaspoon extra-virgin olive oil or 2 teaspoons reserved chickpea brine
- 1 teaspoon smoked paprika
- 1 teaspoon garlic powder

Directions:

1. Preheat the oven to 425°F. Line a baking sheet with parchment paper.
2. After draining the chickpeas, pat dry with a paper towel. Transfer to a medium bowl. Add the olive oil, paprika, and garlic powder. Using a wooden spoon or your hands, toss gently to coat.

3. Spread the chickpeas out on the prepared baking sheet in a single layer. Roast for 30 minutes, rotating the baking sheet after 15 minutes.

4. Turn the oven off, open the oven door about five inches, and allow the chickpeas to cool in the oven. Transfer all of the chickpeas into a glass pint jar or divide evenly among 4 (4-ounce) jelly jars. Cool completely before closing tightly with lids.

Nutrition: Calories: 157 Total fat: 3g Carbohydrates: 28g Fiber: 6g Protein: 6g

30. Tamari Almonds

Preparation Time: 5 minutes

Cooking Time: 15 minutes

Servings: 8

Ingredients:

- 1 pound raw almonds
- 3 tablespoons tamari or soy sauce
- 2 tablespoons extra-virgin olive oil
- 1 tablespoon nutritional yeast
- 1 to 2 teaspoons chili powder, to taste

Directions:

1. Preheat the oven to 400°F. Line a baking sheet with parchment paper.

2. In a medium bowl, combine the almonds, tamari, and olive oil until well coated. Spread the almonds on the prepared baking sheet and roast for 10 to 15 minutes until browned.

3. Cool for 10 minutes, then season with the nutritional yeast and chili powder.

4. Transfer to a glass jar and close tightly with a lid.

Nutrition: Calories: 364 Total fat: 32g Carbohydrates: 13g Fiber: 6g Protein: 13g

31. Taco Pita Pizzas

Preparation Time: 5 minutes

Cooking Time: 7 minutes

Servings: 4

Ingredients:

- 4 sandwich-size pita bread pieces or Sandwich Thins
- 1 cup vegetarian refried beans
- 1 cup pizza sauce
- 1 cup chopped mushrooms
- 1 teaspoon minced jalapeño (optional)

Directions:

1. Preheat the oven to 400°F. Line a large baking sheet with parchment paper.

2. Assemble 4 pizzas: On each pita, spread about ¼ cup of refried beans. Pour ¼ cup of pizza sauce over the beans and spread evenly. Add ¼ cup of mushrooms. Sprinkle ¼ teaspoon of minced jalapeño (if using) over the mushrooms.

3. Place the pizzas on the prepared baking sheet and bake for 7 minutes.

4. Cool completely before placing each pizza in a freezer-safe plastic bag, or store together in one large airtight, freezer-safe container with parchment paper between the pizzas.

Nutrition: Calories: 148 Total fat: 2g Carbohydrates: 29g Fiber: 5g Protein: 6g

32. Risotto Bites

Preparation Time: 15 minutes

Cooking Time: 20 minutes

Servings: 12 bites

Ingredients:

- ½ cup panko bread crumbs

- 1 teaspoon paprika

- 1 teaspoon chipotle powder or ground cayenne pepper

- 1½ cups cold Green Pea Risotto

- Nonstick cooking spray

Directions:

1. Preheat the oven to 425°F. Line a baking sheet with parchment paper.

2. On a large plate, combine the panko, paprika, and chipotle powder. Set aside.

3. Roll 2 tablespoons of the risotto into a ball. Gently roll in the bread crumbs and place on the prepared baking sheet. Repeat to make a total of 12 balls.

4. Spritz the tops of the risotto bites with nonstick cooking spray and bake for 15 to 20 minutes, until they begin to brown.

5. Cool completely before storing in a large airtight container in a single layer (add a piece of parchment paper for a second layer) or in a plastic freezer bag.

Nutrition: Calories: 100 Total fat: 2g Carbohydrates: 17g Fiber: 5g Protein: 6g

33. Healthy Protein Bars

Preparation Time: 19 minutes

Cooking Time: 0 minutes

Servings: 12 balls

Ingredients:

- 1 large banana
- 1 cup of rolled oats
- 1 serving of vegan vanilla protein powder

Directions:

1. Using your food processor, blend the protein powder, and rolled oats.

2. Blend them for 1 minute until you have a semi-coarse mixture. The oats should be slightly chopped, but not powdered.

3. Add the banana and form a pliable and coarse dough.

4. Shape into either balls or small bars and store them in a container.

5. Eat one and store the rest in an airtight container in the refrigerator!

Nutrition: Fat 0.7 g Carbohydrates 8 g Protein- 2.7 g Calories: 47

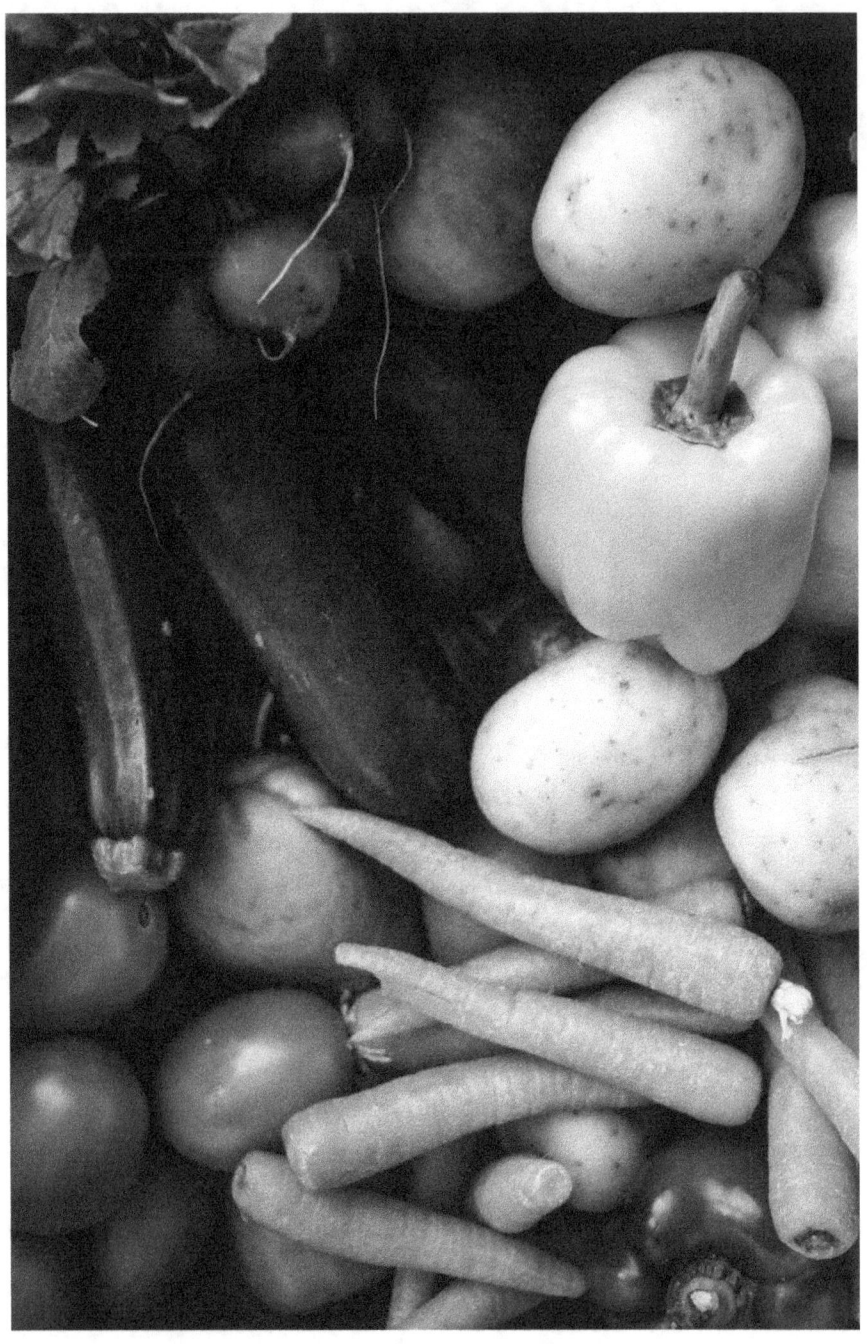

CHAPTER 7:

JUICES AND SMOOTHIES RECIPES

34. Mango Smoothie

Preparation Time: 3 minutes

Cooking Time: 0 minutes

Servings: 2

Ingredients:

- 2 fresh mangoes
- 1 frozen banana
- 1/2 cup milk
- 1/2 cup yogurt

- ⅛ Cup unsweetened coconut

Directions:

1. Put everything into the blender until the desired consistency is achieved. Enjoy immediately!

Nutrition: Calories: 329.6 Carbohydrates: 64.5g Protein: 6.3g Fat: 8.6g Sodium: 27.7mg Fiber: 7.2g Sugar: 53.1g

35. Beetroot Smoothie

Preparation Time: 4 minutes

Cooking Time: 0 minutes

Servings: 1

Ingredients:

- ½ apple (e.g., Golden Delicious)
- 1 small beetroot, pre-cooked
- ½ lime (juiced)
- 1 tsp. maple syrup
- 10 mint, fresh, and 1¼ cups water

Directions:

1. Put everything into the blender. Enjoy!

Directions: Calories: 95 Fat: 1g Cholesterol: 2mg Carbohydrates: 19g Fiber: 4g Sugar: 13g Protein: 4g

36. Avocado Smoothie

Preparation Time: 5 minutes

Cooking Time: 0 minutes

Servings: 2

Ingredients:

- ½ avocado
- 3 celery stalks
- 1 lime
- Fresh mint leaves
- 1 tsp. linseeds

Directions:

1. Put everything into the blender. Enjoy!
2. Better when it's cool, you can keep the smoothie in the refrigerator for 1 to 2 days in an airtight container.

Nutrition: Calories: 178 Sugar: 8g Sodium: 105mg Fat: 11.6g Saturated fat: 2.1g Carbohydrates: 19.3g Fiber: 5.7g Protein: 2.5g

37. Red Smoothie

Preparation Time: 5 minutes

Cooking Time: 0 minutes

Servings: 1

Ingredients:

- 2 cups mixed frozen red berries such as strawberries and raspberries
- 1 small red beet, peeled and thinly sliced
- 1 tablespoon fresh lemon juice
- 1 tablespoon honey
- 2 teaspoons unrefined extra-virgin coconut oil

Directions:

1. Put everything into the blender until the desired consistency is achieved. Enjoy immediately!

Nutrition: Calories: 221 Fat: 1g Cholesterol: 0mg Sodium: 10mg Carbohydrates: 56g Fiber: 12g Sugar: 33g Protein: 3g

38. Kale Smoothie

Preparation Time: 3 minutes

Cooking Time: 0 minutes

Servings: 1

Ingredients:

- 2 cups of kale leaves
- 1 cup of almond milk
- 1 banana
- 1 apple
- Cinnamon

Directions:

1. Put everything into the blender. Enjoy!
2. You may need a lid and scrape the blender walls to blend everything together. Pour into a glass and serve immediately!

Nutrition: Calories: 187 Fat: 9g Cholesterol: 3mg Sodium: 149mg Carbohydrates: 27g Fiber: 4g Sugar: 13g Protein: 8g

39. Melon Smoothie

Preparation Time: 5 minutes

Cooking Time: 0 minutes

Servings: 2

Ingredients:

- 1/4 cantaloupe - peeled, seeded, and cubed
- 1/4 honeydew melon - peeled, seeded, and cubed
- 1 lime, juiced
- 3 fresh mint leaves
- 2 tablespoons sugar

Directions:

1. Combine cantaloupe, honeydew, lime juice, and sugar in a blender. Blend until smooth. Pour into glasses and serve.

Nutrition: Calories: 70 Fat: 0.2g Carbohydrates: 18.1g Protein: 0.8g Cholesterol: 0mg Sodium: 20mg

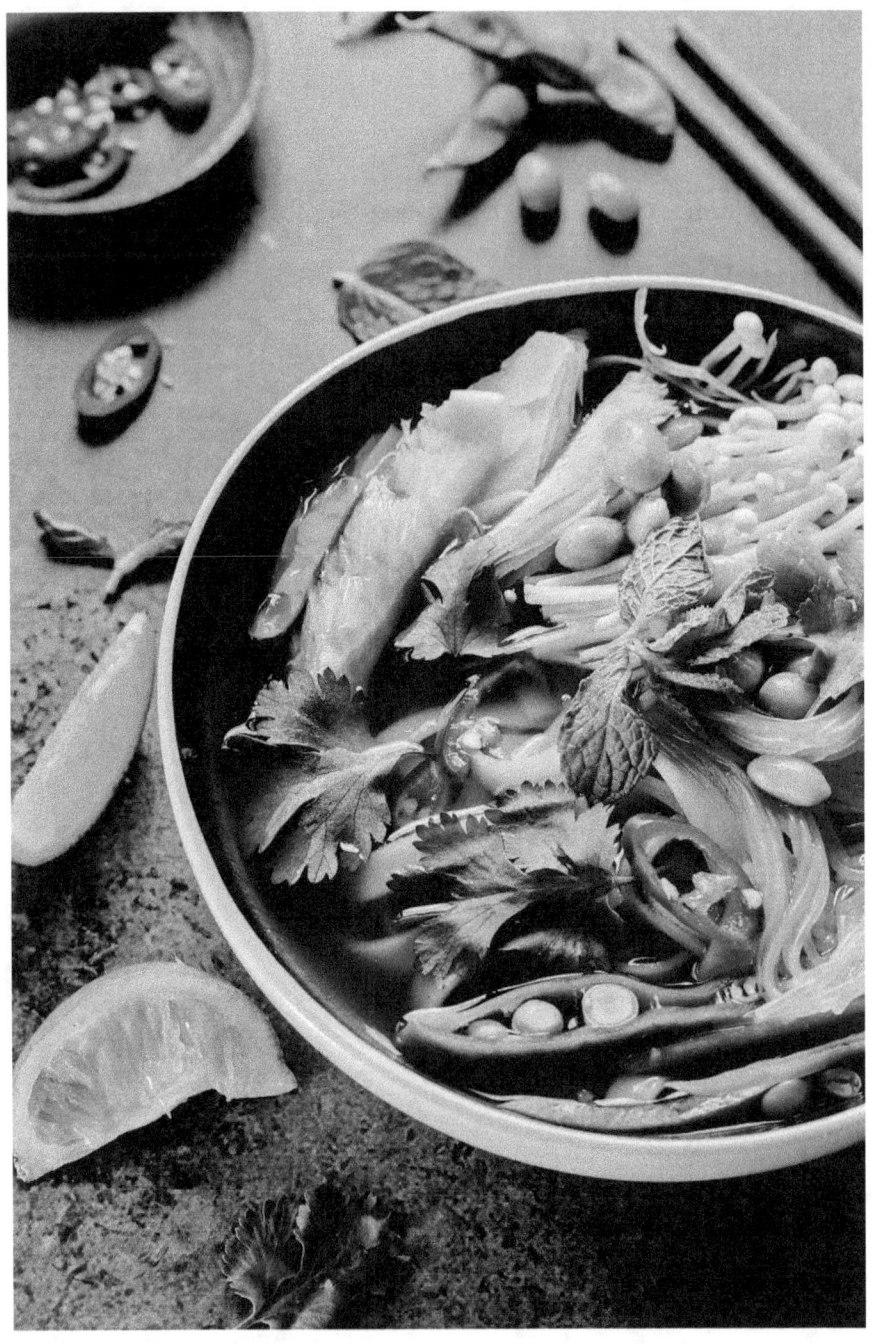

CHAPTER 8:

OTHER RECIPES

40. Cauliflower Mash

Preparation Time: 15 Minutes

Cooking Time: 12 minutes

Servings: 3

Ingredients:

- 1 head cauliflower, chopped
- 2 tablespoons homemade vegetable broth
- 2 garlic cloves, chopped
- 2 tablespoons coconut oil
- Salt, as required

Directions:

1. In a microwave-safe bowl, add the cauliflower and broth and microwave on High for about 10-12 minutes.

2. In a food processor, add the cauliflower mixture and remaining ingredients and pulse until smooth.

3. Serve immediately.

Nutrition: Calories: 104 Fats: 9.2g Carbs: 5.5g Proteins: 1.9g

41. Apple Leather

Preparation Time: 15 Minutes

Cooking Time: 12 hours 25 minutes

Servings: 2

Ingredients:

- 1 cup water
- 8 cups apples, peeled, cored and chopped
- 1 tablespoon ground cinnamon
- 2 tablespoons fresh lemon juice

Directions:

1. In a large pan, add water and apples over medium-low heat and simmer for about 10-15 minutes, stirring occasionally.
2. Remove from heat and set aside to cool slightly.
3. In a blender, add apple mixture and pulse until smooth.
4. Return the mixture into the pan over medium-low heat.
5. Stir in cinnamon and lemon juice and simmer for about 10 minutes.

6. Transfer the mixture onto dehydrator trays, and with the back of the spoon smooth the top.

7. Set the dehydrator at 135 degrees F.

8. Dehydrate for about 10-12 hours.

9. Cut the apple leather into equal-sized rectangles.

10. Now, roll each rectangle to make fruit rolls.

Nutrition: Calories: 238 Fats: 0.9g Carbs: 63.1g Proteins: 1.3g

42. Sautéed Brussels Sprout

Preparation Time: 15 minutes

Cooking Time: 15 minutes

Servings: 2

Ingredients:

- ½ pound Brussels sprouts, halved
- 1 tablespoon olive oil
- 2 garlic cloves, minced
- ½ teaspoon red pepper flakes, crushed
- Salt and ground black pepper, as required
- 1 tablespoon fresh lemon juice

Directions:

1. Arrange a steamer basket over a large pan of boiling water.
2. Place the asparagus in a steamer basket. Cover and steam for about 6 to 8 minutes. Drain well.
3. In a large skillet, heat oil over medium heat.
4. Add garlic and red pepper flakes and sauté for about 1 minute.

5. Add the Brussels sprouts, salt, and black pepper, and sauté for 4-5 minutes.

6. Stir in the lemon juice and sauté for 1 minute more.

7. Serve hot.

Nutrition: Calories: 117 Fats: 7.6g Carbs: 11.7g Proteins: 4.2g

43. Green Beans with Mushrooms

Preparation Time: 15 Minutes

Cooking Time: 20 minutes

Servings: 2

Ingredients:

- 2 tablespoons olive oil
- 2 tablespoons yellow onion, minced
- ½ teaspoon garlic, minced
- 1 (8-ounce) package white mushrooms, sliced
- 1 cup frozen green beans
- Salt and ground black pepper, as required

Directions:

1. In a skillet, heat the oil over medium heat and sauté the onion and garlic for about 1 minute. Add the mushrooms and cook for about 6-7 minutes.

2. Stir in the green beans and cook for about 5-10 minutes or until desired doneness.

3. Serve hot.

Nutrition: Calories: 166 Fats: 14.4g Carbs: 8.8g Proteins: 4.7g

44. Pinto Beans with Salsa

Preparation Time: 15 minutes

Cooking Time: 12 minutes

Servings: 4

Ingredients:

- 1 tablespoon canola oil
- 1 small onion, chopped
- 1 garlic clove, minced
- 2 teaspoons fresh cilantro, minced
- 2 (15-ounce) cans pinto beans, rinsed and drained
- 2/3 cup salsa

Directions:

1. In a large skillet, heat the oil over medium heat and sauté the onion for about 4-5 minutes.
2. Add the garlic and cilantro and sauté for about 1 minute.
3. Stir in the beans and salsa and cook for about 4-5 minutes or until heated completely.

4. Serve hot.

Nutrition: Calories: 182 Fats: 4.3g Carbs: 26.4g Proteins: 8.2g

45. Asparagus Soup

Preparation Time: 15 minutes

Cooking Time: 40 minutes

Servings: 4

Ingredients:

- 1 tablespoon olive oil
- 3 scallions, chopped
- 1½ pounds fresh asparagus, trimmed and chopped
- 4 cups homemade vegetable broth
- 2 tablespoons fresh lemon juice
- Salt and ground black pepper, as required

Directions:

In a large pan, heat the oil over medium heat and sauté the scallion for about 4-5 minutes.

Stir in the asparagus and broth and bring to a boil.

Reduce the heat to low and simmer, covered for about 25-30 minutes.

Remove from the heat and set aside to cool slightly.

Now, transfer the soup into a high-speed blender in 2 batches and pulse until smooth.

Return the soup into the same pan over medium heat and simmer for about 4-5 minutes.

Stir in the lemon juice, salt, and black pepper and remove from the heat. Serve hot.

Nutrition: Calories: 84 Fats: 3.8g Carbs: 10.6g Proteins: 4g

46. Beet Soup

Preparation Time: 10 minutes

Cooking Time: 5 minutes

Servings: 2

Ingredients:

2 cups coconut yogurt

4 teaspoons fresh lemon juice

2 cups beets, trimmed, peeled and chopped

2 tablespoons fresh dill

Salt, as required

Directions:

In a high-speed blender, add all ingredients and pulse until smooth.

Transfer the soup into a pan over medium heat and cook for about 3-5 minutes or until heated through.

Serve immediately.

Nutrition: Calories: 255 Fats: 11.5g Carbs: 29.9g Proteins: 15.6g

47. Pears in Red Wine Sauce

Preparation Time: 10 minutes Cooking Time: 10 minutes

Servings: 6

Ingredients:

6 pears

1 cup of superfine sugar

1 wine glass of red wine (5-6 oz.)

1 pinch cinnamon

1 vanilla pod

1 clove bud

Directions:

Peel the pears.

In a pressure cooker pot, dissolve the sugar in the wine together with vanilla and clove.

Place the pears into the pot and close the lid.

Cook for 7 minutes on low heat.

Nutrition: Total Carbs 66.7 g Fat 0.5 g Protein 0.8g Calories 277

48. Polenta

Preparation Time: 5 minutes

Cooking Time: 15 minutes

Servings: 6

Ingredients:

1 cup polenta (coarse-ground cornmeal)

4 cups vegetable broth

3–4 tsp. butter

½ cup Mexican blend shredded cheese

¼ cup half and half

Salt to taste

Directions:

Press the "Sauté" function on the Instant Pot. Add the broth and polenta, whisk together.

When it starts to boil, seal the lid. Select "Manual" and set on high pressure for 7 minutes.

When the cooking cycle is finished, release the pressure naturally.

Use a whisk to blend in the butter, cheese, and half and half. It will help to thicken the polenta.

Salt, if needed, and serve.

Nutrition: Calories 170 Total Carbs 22 g Fat 6 g Protein 5 g

49. Carrots in Thyme

Preparation Time: 10 minutes Cooking Time: 5 minutes

Servings: 4

Ingredients

4 carrots, peeled

1½ tsp. fresh thyme

2 Tbsp. butter

½ cup water

1 dash salt

Directions:

Melt butter in the pressure cooker over medium heat.

Cut the peeled carrots into sticks (like French fries).

Add the carrots, thyme, salt, and ½ cup of water to the pot.

Cover and cook at high pressure for 1 minutes, then turn off the heat and let sit for 4 min.

Release the pressure gently. Serve.

Nutrition: Total Carbs 6 g Fat 5.8 g Protein 0.6 g Calories 77

50. Smoky Pecan Brussels sprouts

Preparation Time: 5 minutes

Cooking Time: 10 minutes

Servings: 2

Ingredients:

2 cups small baby Brussels sprouts

¼ cup water

½ tsp. liquid smoke

¼ cup pecans, chopped

2 Tbsps. maple syrup

Salt and pepper to taste

Directions:

Add water, Brussels sprouts, and liquid smoke to an Instant Pot, mix well.

Lock the lid and close the pressure valve. Cook on high pressure for 2 minutes.

When the cooking time is up, release the pressure manually.

Select the "Sauté" function and add the pecans and maple syrup. Reduce the liquid as you finish cooking the sprouts. Once the sprouts are tender, remove from the heat.

Salt and pepper to taste and serve.

Nutrition: Calories 113 Total Carbs 17 g Fat 3 g Protein 5 g

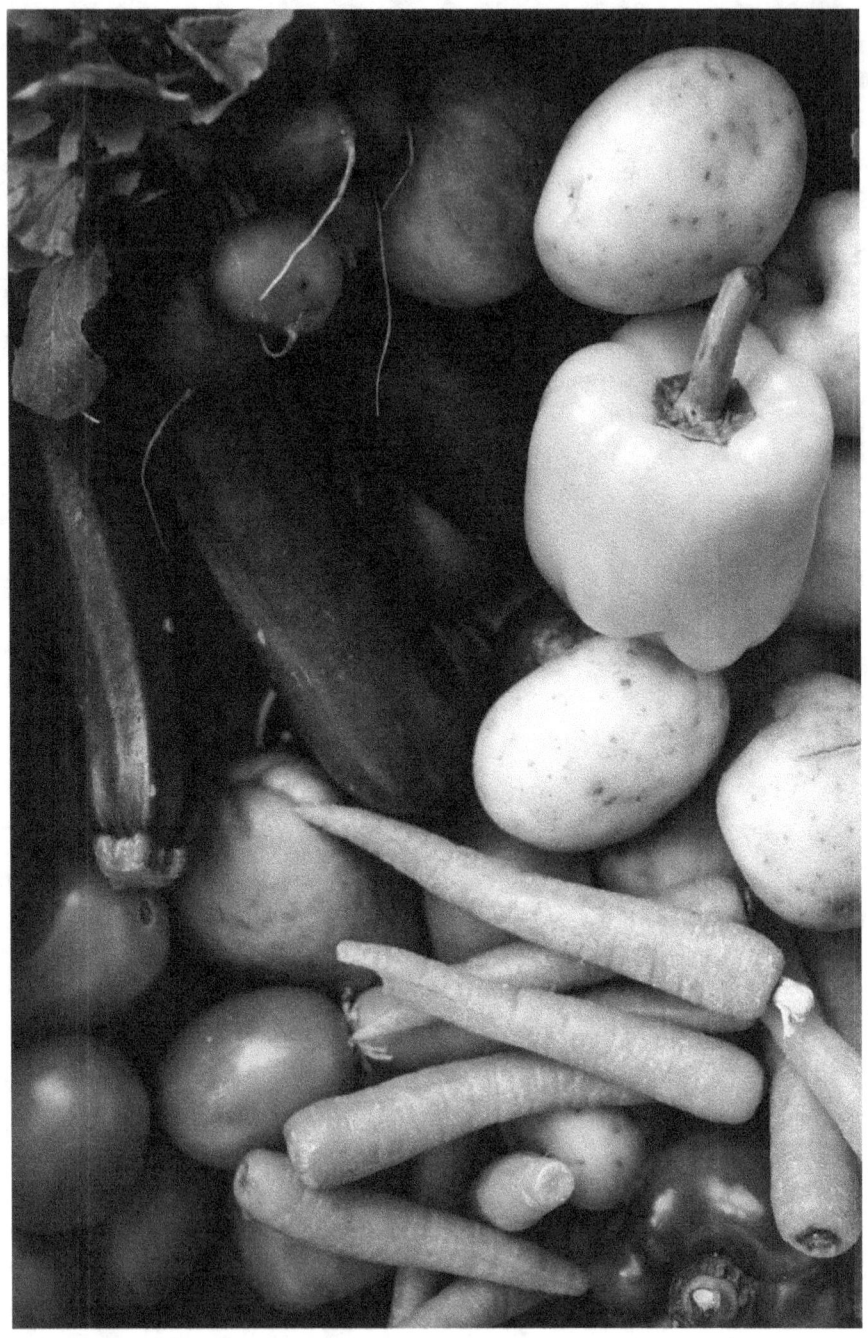

CONCLUSION

Well done! Thank you for reaching the end of this book, The Complete Vegetarian Cookbook.

Hopefully, this book has helped you understand that making vegetarian recipes and diet easier can improve your life, not only by improving your health and helping you lose weight, but also by saving you money and time.

Remember that vegetarianism is a choice, not a religion.

Be flexible when it comes to your diet and enjoy new tastes and experiences.

Don't be afraid of meat substitutes, but experiment with using them sparingly. There is no need to completely replace meat with fake meat products like tofu or processed soy-based vegetarian burgers and hot dogs. Not only are they expensive, but fake meats contain artificial ingredients that may or may not be healthy for you.

Also, if you are not used to eating a vegetarian diet, start with a few vegetarian meals and snacks during the week, and see how you feel.

You can always add more vegetarian meals to your diet later. It is better to be even slightly vegetarians than completely non-vegetarian.

The best tip I can give you about making vegetarian recipes is to experiment and have fun!

Here are some more tips to help you with your vegetarian diet:

1. Remember that vegetarianism is not a destination, it is a journey.

2. A vegetarian diet is plant-based. This means that you should try to eat more plants and less animal products. You should also be careful not to replace whole foods with their processed counterparts, such as replacing whole foods such as fruits and vegetables with fruit juice and pasta sauce.

3. Try to avoid processed food whenever possible, while still maintaining your balanced diet and nutrients that you need for your health. An easier way of doing this will be to make your own food when

possible and try to avoid packaged, pre-prepared foods at the grocery store.

4. Avoid processed food products that contain artificial ingredients, such as sweeteners, colors, and flavors.

5. Avoid highly processed meat substitutes. Remember to use meat substitutes in moderation or as an occasional treat.

6. If you choose to eat meat substitutes such as tofu, be sure to thoroughly cook it and try different ways of preparing it

7. You may need to gradually introduce your family and friends to your new eating habits. Don't expect everyone to support you or enjoy the same things you do when it comes to vegetarian recipes. As long as you are happy with your food choices, that is the most important thing – even if it means making some changes at home!

When you are having a hard time, always remember this: You can always choose to stop being a vegetarian.

You can simply start eating meat again if you are struggling with your new diet.

Remember that it is okay to be a part-time vegetarian, but if you find that you cannot maintain the lifestyle or are unhappy with your choice, it is always better to go back to eating a non-veg diet.

There is no shame in making changes to your vegetarian recipe routine if you need to, and you will not shame yourself for deciding that a strict vegetarian diet does not work for you.

I know that there are many books and choosing my book is amazing. I am thankful that you stopped and took the time to decide. You made a great decision, and I am sure that you enjoyed it.

I will be even happier if you will add some comments. Feedbacks helped by growing, and they still do. They help me to choose better content and new ideas. So, maybe your feedback can trigger an idea for my next book. Thank you again for downloading this book!

I hope you enjoyed reading my book!

www.ingramcontent.com/pod-product-compliance
Lightning Source LLC
Chambersburg PA
CBHW070937080526
44589CB00013B/1547